Jéssica Moraes de Araujo
Irineu Sousa Junior
Rayane C. Moura

Health Literacy of Elderly People with Hypertension and/or Diabetes

Jéssica Moraes de Araujo
Irineu Sousa Junior
Rayane C. Moura

Health Literacy of Elderly People with Hypertension and/or Diabetes

A Study with the Elderly in Oeiras - Piauí

ScienciaScripts

Imprint

Any brand names and product names mentioned in this book are subject to trademark, brand or patent protection and are trademarks or registered trademarks of their respective holders. The use of brand names, product names, common names, trade names, product descriptions etc. even without a particular marking in this work is in no way to be construed to mean that such names may be regarded as unrestricted in respect of trademark and brand protection legislation and could thus be used by anyone.

Cover image: www.ingimage.com

This book is a translation from the original published under ISBN 978-613-9-72395-9.

Publisher:
Sciencia Scripts
is a trademark of
Dodo Books Indian Ocean Ltd. and OmniScriptum S.R.L publishing group

120 High Road, East Finchley, London, N2 9ED, United Kingdom
Str. Armeneasca 28/1, office 1, Chisinau MD-2012, Republic of Moldova, Europe
Printed at: see last page
ISBN: 978-620-7-73960-8

JÉSSICA MORAES DE ARAUJO
FEDERAL UNIVERSITY OF PIAUÍ

IRINEU DE SOUSA JÚNIOR
FEDERAL INSTITUTE OF PIAUÍ

RAYANE CARVALHO DE MOURA
FEDERAL UNIVERSITY OF PIAUÍ

EVALUATION OF THE HEALTH LITERACY OF ELDERLY PEOPLE WITH HYPERTENSION AND/OR DIABETES IN OEIRAS- PIAUÍ

SUMMARY

INTRODUCTION: The WHO considers health literacy to be one of the most important factors in determining a society's state of health. People with low health literacy will find it difficult to understand and follow instructions provided by health specialists. In Brazil, schooling levels and functional literacy rates remain very low in some areas and in subgroups of the Brazilian population. **OBJECTIVE:** This study investigated the level of health literacy among elderly individuals with hypertension and/or diabetes in the city of Oeiras-Piauí. **METHODOLOGY:** A validated SAHLPA instrument was used, consisting of 50 items that assessed the individual's ability to correctly pronounce and understand common medical terms. The sample consisted of 100 elderly residents of the city of Oeiras Piauí who attended the Basic Health Units and/or the Better Age Club, aged > 60 years, hypertensive and/or diabetic, self-reported ability to read and speak Portuguese; no diagnosis of dementia; no visual impairment or hearing problems. **RESULTS AND DISCUSSION:** All the study participants had completed some level of schooling and the SAHLPA-50 showed that 92% of the elderly had inadequate health literacy according to their answers to the questionnaire. **FINAL CONSIDERATIONS:** It was possible to investigate that the level of health literacy is very low, in other words, an unsatisfactory level. These conditions depend on a whole change in the system in which we live, in addition to promoting the experience of science by inserting technical and scientific terms where such activities should reduce the difficulties of access. **KEYWORDS:** Health Literacy, Reading, Health Promotion, Health Education.

CONTENTS

1 INTRODUCTION

Reading is understood as an act that arises from mediation, the act of deciphering signs that translate a language. It's not just about understanding the world through the prism of an author, but also capturing that language that is expressed through signs and that can make communicative action fluid. Reading is also a dynamic process of learning, of mediation with: patterns and codes (RECIIS, 2009).

Health literacy is defined in the Institute of Medicine report (2004) as a recipe for ending confusion as "the degree to which individuals have the ability to obtain, process, and understand information and services needed to make health appropriate". It is a determining factor in health knowledge, health behaviour, healthcare use and disease progression (PARKER; RATZAN; LURIE, 2003) (SUDORE; YAFFE; SATTERFIELD et al, 2006).

The concept of health literacy is not a recent one, and Simonds (1974) is credited with first using the terms together in the 1970s to refer to the need for health education in a school context (RATZAN, 2001; BERNHARDT; BROWNFIELD; PARKER, 2005).

The World Health Organisation (WHO) considers health literacy to be one of the most important factors in determining a society's state of health and calls on countries around the world to create a community for health literacy.
coordination of strategic activities involving the promotion of health education (REISI et al, 2011).

Low health literacy is related to perceived low self-efficacy in preventing and managing health problems, as well as ineffective health behaviours: inappropriate use of medication, overuse of health services, or ineffectiveness in dealing with emergency situations (ZARCADOOLAS; PLEASANT; GREER, 2006). Health literacy involves learning information about health issues and the ability to understand and use this information. There is a close relationship between health literacy and quality of life (TEERÃ, 2012).

People with low health literacy will struggle to understand and follow instructions provided by health specialists, incur additional medical costs, have poorer health, higher rates of hospitalisation and emergency department use, and use less preventive care (TEHRANI-BANIHASHEMI et al, 2007). There is a lot of evidence that people with low health literacy (including numeracy in health) are less able to understand the contents of information leaflets on food or drugs (ROTHMAN et al, 2006) and are less able to navigate health systems (BAKER et al, 2008).

In Brazil, despite the progress made towards universal basic education in recent decades, schooling levels and functional literacy rates remain very low in some areas and in subgroups of the Brazilian population. A recent cross-sectional study carried out in 204 cities showed that 27 per cent of elderly Brazilians reported being illiterate and an additional 22 per cent reported basic reading and writing problems (APOLINÁRIO et al, 2012).

Several years of formal education alone is not a reliable indicator of health literacy and individuals with low health literacy skills may try to hide it, it is difficult to recognise those patients with inadequate health literacy during routine clinical care (KELLY; HAIDET, 2007). Developing valid and reliable health literacy through instruments is extremely important, as they help healthcare providers to identify patients who may require special communication needs and benefit from specific interventions in clinical settings (APOLINÁRIO et al, 2012).

In any case, Osvaldo Santos (2010) said that in the last ten years there has been a considerable research effort to develop instruments that are valid for measuring this latent variable and sensitive enough to detect differences (when they exist), both between population groups and within groups (for example, in longitudinal designs).

However, agreement has not yet been reached on the criteria to be used to select the most appropriate measure of health literacy for different groups (POWERS; TRINH; BOSWORTH, 2010). Measurement selection can be particularly important in healthcare settings, where the importance of patient understanding of health management is essential. The issue of measurement selection is especially important with older adults, where the substantial variation in educational attainment and interactions with healthcare across the lifespan raises concerns about the duration and complexity of health literacy tools (FEDERMAN et al, 2009).

An equal and sustainable healthcare plan is not complete without the skills needed to make appropriate health-related decisions. More high-quality research is needed to develop evidence-based interactive health literacy programmes targeted specifically at older adults and to evaluate the use of standardised health literacy research tools (MANAFO, 2012).

Low health literacy is therefore an important risk factor for the onset of numerous morbidities. Therefore, the aim of this article is to investigate the level of health literacy among elderly individuals with hypertension and/or diabetes in the city of Oeiras-Piauí, so that the root of the problem can be diagnosed, interventions can be made and the associated complications can be minimised, thus improving health systems.

2 THEORETICAL FRAMEWORK

2.1 HEALTH PROMOTION

Health promotion emerged as an international "new conception of health" in the mid-1970s, as a result of the debate in the previous decade on the social and economic determination of health and the construction of a conception that was not centred on disease (HEIDMANN et al, 2006). The modern health promotion movement emerged in Canada in May 1974, with the publication of what is known as the "Lalonde Report", which was politically, technically and economically motivated to tackle the rising cost of healthcare (LALONDE, 1974). It was the first official document to be labelled health promotion. It was based on the concept of the "health field" and introduced the so-called "determinants of health".

The Lalonde report advocates that health actions should aim to add years to life and to add life to years, in other words, to guarantee the quality of life of individuals and groups. An important concept is that of the health field - a set of practices and knowledge that influence health and go beyond health services - which underpins the proposal for an explanatory health model, a kind of map of the territory in which the role of four groups in determining the health-disease process is highlighted: human biology (genetics and human function), the organisation of health services; the environment (natural and social) and lifestyle (individual behaviour that affects health) (CARVALHO, 2004).

Thus, in the mid-1980s, an alternative promotion discourse began to emerge and, in 1984, the WHO/Europe produced a preliminary document containing the key elements of the new health promotion, reinforcing the notion of the social determination of health (MINISTÉRIO DA SAÚDE, 2002; CARVALHO, 2002). That same year, the *Beyond Health Care* Conference was held in Toronto, Canada, which laid the foundations for the healthy cities movement (BUSS; 2003; CARVALHO, 2002; PANAMERICAN HEALTH ORGANISATION, 1995). In 1985, WHO/Europe published the 38 goals for health in the European region and (CZERESNIA, 2003) in 1986, the *Health City Movement* document was published, and this discourse found expression in Canada (CZERESNIA, 2003; BUSS, 2000).

The First International Conference on Health Promotion organised by the WHO in 1986, the Ottawa Charter (generally recognised as the founding framework for health promotion as an institutional field of practice and reflection on public health) states that in order to achieve a state of complete physical, mental and social well-being, an individual or group must be able to identify and fulfil aspirations, satisfy needs and transform or deal with environments. Health is therefore seen as a resource for everyday life, not the goal of life. It is a positive concept emphasising social and personal resources as well as physical capabilities. Therefore, health promotion is not just the responsibility of one sector and goes beyond healthy lifestyles to well-being (WHO, 1986; SANCHEZ; CICONELLI, 2012).

The persistence of the old regime, which is intertwined with the new one, democracy, is reflected in the attitudes of the majority of the population, who maintain a posture of submission to the power of a few, whose aim is to preserve this situation, that is, to maintain power. This is the great resistance to be overcome, because Health Promotion considers that better living conditions and health can only be achieved through the active participation of the population, which presupposes a more horizontal and less submissive relationship. In other words, Health Promotion wants situations of paternalism and assistance to be avoided through the effective participation of the population and for effective political mechanisms to begin to promote equity in the different regions of the country (BYDLOWSKI; PEREIRA; WESTPHAL, 2004).

Changes in the field of public health, in particular the creation of the health promotion movement, have led to fundamental changes in the principles that have underpinned health education for some time. In the 'old' public health, health education had a single focus: disease prevention. The 'new' health education must go beyond the biomedical conceptualisation of health and encompass broader objectives, since health is no longer just the absence of disease, but a source of life. Thus, in its contemporary version, health education is no longer just aimed at preventing illness, but at preparing the individual to fight for a healthier life. In this new paradigm, the individual must be encouraged to make decisions about their own life, a notion of autonomy that creates an ideal of self-government. In the same way as health promotion, neoliberalism, a new form of political rationality that has predominated in contemporary Western societies, defends the thesis of investing in autonomy and individual choice (OLIVEIRA, 2005).

Integrating preventive, promotional and care actions; integrating professionals in interdisciplinary and multi-professional teams for a more comprehensive understanding of health problems and more effective interventions; integrating parts of a living organism, torn apart and objectified by the reductionist view of biomedicine, and recognising in it a subject, similar to myself; this implies assimilating the principle of integrality in favour of reorienting the care model. This assimilation must take place on a daily basis in the encounters between professionals and users in the health services, where rationalities are exercised, whether they are to maintain the current hegemonic model of care - markedly reductionist, biologicist, individualist, centred on the disease and oriented towards a cure - or to build a new model of care - comprehensive, humanised and committed to meeting the needs and guaranteeing the population's right to health (ALVES, 2005).

Health promotion is an important response as it highlights intersectoral actions as a strategy for tackling environmental problems, urbanisation, food and nutritional security, unemployment, housing, the use of licit and illicit drugs, etc. (CAMPOS et al, 2004).

To talk about health promotion in Brazil, which is inseparable from reflecting on the creation of the Unified Health System and our ongoing struggle to improve it, is also to talk about a reality of historical inequities of great proportions, which pose daily challenges not only to the health sector, but to all those who build public policies. It means remembering and exercising our anthropophagic stance, it means asking, in view of our ethical commitment to caring for the health of individuals and communities, how we think about health promotion here and what it can do to help us generate other modes of health care and management, of creating life and other realities (CAMPOS et al, 2004).

Health promotion has exerted a growing influence on the organisation of the health system in various countries and regions of the world. Since international and regional conferences have been held, there has been a progressive but also contradictory evolution of its premises and strategies. These contradictions stem from the various conceptions of health promotion, which can be grouped into two large groups: behavioural, or lifestyle changes, and those that seek to articulate the theme of health with the theme of living conditions and quality of life (BUSS, 2003).

It is within the scope of health promotion to invest in the education of citizens and to work towards the establishment of truly democratic spaces, especially at local level, in order to develop policies that are based on identified health problems and needs and that can be continually evaluated and revised on this basis. The dissemination of information and education are bases for decision-making and important components of health promotion, a concern that seems to be linked to the principle of empowerment, understood as the process of enabling individuals and communities to take greater control over the personal, socio-economic and environmental factors that affect health (WHO, 1998). According to Labonte (1996b), the term refers to the process of transforming the feeling of powerlessness internalised by individuals in the face of power inequalities. The first step towards community empowerment "is to give back the power to define" (LABONTE, 1996a), which would be fundamental to community health promotion, since communities are responsible for defining and choosing their priority problems and needs.

It is important to emphasise that when implementing health promotion policies, the principles of empowerment and participation should not be separated. The WHO itself (WHO, 1986) recognises that guaranteeing access to information and expanding health knowledge without increasing the capacity for control and prospects for change only contributes to generating anxiety and fostering a sense of powerlessness. It is therefore essential to overcome the barriers that limit the exercise of democracy and develop flexible systems that reinforce social participation and citizenship, as advocated by the International Conferences held, especially those in Ottawa and Bogotá (SÍCOLI; NASCIMENTO, 2003).

The great challenge of health promotion, especially in the Latin American context, is to change the scenario in which enormous social inequality still prevails, with deteriorating living conditions for the majority of the population, along with increased health risks and fewer resources to deal with them. The fight for health is equivalent to improving quality of life (income, education, transport, leisure, housing and others) and should be part of the main health promotion strategies (HEIDMANN et al, 2006).

The emergence of the New Public Health signals a considerable expansion of the field of action of health promotion. In the name of the absolute eradication of risks, the environment is scrutinised in its physical, psychological and social dimensions, consequently multiplying the objects to be measured, monitored and regulated. On the basis of calculating probability, the range of interventions and prescriptions expanded, and they were deduced and justified on the basis of the fact that, in order to be suspect, a person does not need to show symptoms of danger or abnormality, but simply possess the characteristic that the experts responsible for prevention policies classify as a "risk factor" (CARVALHO,

2004).

What Health Promotion proposes is action to reverse situations such as those described, so that equity can be achieved, i.e. opportunities can be created for social justice, in which biological differences and free choice are respected, while at the same time ensuring minimum conditions for dignified survival (BYDLOWSKI; PEREIRA; WESTPHAL, 2004).

More than risk factors, health promotion is called upon to deal with complex situations where risk is no longer external to the individual, but is part of a unique complex of multiple dimensions - biological, social and cultural (CARVALHO, 2004).

However, it is important to recognise that most professionals are still unaware of the true meaning of health promotion. There is confusion between the concepts of promotion and prevention, the behavioural approach of lifestyle changes predominates, and health is still understood as the absence of disease. In view of this, for health services to promote health, professionals need to understand and broaden their vision of health promotion, including themselves as critical players and participants in the process of building and reformulating this system (HEIDMANN et al, 2006).

To this end, a National Health Promotion Policy will be more effective to the extent that it builds actions in terms of lifestyles that rely on people's ability to self-regulate without this meaning that the state has to take away its responsibilities in terms of living conditions and, at the same time, work to formulate legislation that makes it more difficult to be exposed to risk situations, reducing the population's vulnerability. We are therefore betting on the articulation of the concepts of health promotion and harm reduction to create other ways of working between respect for individual choices and a commitment to collective health. Thinking about harm reduction means thinking about a way of dealing with risks that doesn't mean giving up our technical, clinical and epidemiological knowledge and, at the same time, doesn't mean imprisoning life in disciplinary and hygienist mechanisms

(CAMPOS et al, 2004).

Initially, it is necessary to take on the process of Health Promotion as a change in focus, concepts and ways of working, with the aim of overcoming the fragmentation and hyper-specialisation that exists today in the Western world, i.e. all areas of knowledge becoming increasingly specialised in understanding the infinitely small, as Carvalho (2003) comments. The same author also observes that, despite the efforts of some areas of knowledge, scientific culture still remains distant from the humanities, and minimising this distance so that they move in the same direction, challenging and breaking down barriers, progressing towards planetary sustainability, should be the purpose of society.

2.2 HEALTH EDUCATION

Due to its magnitude, health education should be seen as an important aspect of prevention, and in practice it should be concerned with improving the living conditions and health of the population. Considering that health education is related to learning, designed to achieve health, it is necessary for it to be geared towards serving the population according to their reality. This is because health education should provoke conflict in individuals, creating the opportunity for people to think and rethink their culture, and to transform their own reality (OLIVEIRA; GONÇALVES, 2004).

Education is present at all times in the lives of human beings. It involves interaction between the people involved in the educational context and between them and the world around them, with the aim of changing both (GIRONDI; NOTHAFT; MALLMANN, 2006). However, it is a complex process and there is no single definition.

In the specific case of health education, it can be said that its concepts and purposes have adapted according to the paradigm shifts that have taken place in the health sector and have also been influenced by the transformations that have taken place in the pedagogical processes of school education in general (MACIEL, 2008).

As an area of knowledge, it requires an embodied vision of different sciences, both education and health, integrating disciplines such as psychology, sociology, philosophy and anthropology (MACHADO et al., 2007).

Traditionally, health education, initially called Sanitary Education, arose in Brazil from the need of the Brazilian state to control the epidemics of infectious diseases that threatened the country's agro-export economy during the Old Republic at the beginning of the 20th century (MACIEL, 2009).

Health education has undergone constant changes. First called health education, it was limited to activities aimed at publishing books, leaflets and catalogues which were distributed in companies and schools, but it was inefficient as it was unable to reach all sections of society (OLIVEIRA; GONÇALVES, 2004). Around the 1970s, what was then known as health education became health education, and it is important to note that more than a change in terminology, a new concept in health promotion began with the aim of introducing the health programmes developed by the Ministry and the State Health Departments (LEVY et al, 2003).

Around the 1970s, health education in Brazil was basically an initiative of the political and economic elites, centred on their own interests. Then, under the military regime, health policy was geared towards the expansion of private medical services, mainly hospitals, so educational activities had no place. With the conquest of political democracy and the construction of the Unified Health System in the 1980s, social movements began to fight for more global changes in social and health policies (VASCONCELOS, 1998).

Regardless of the socio-economic component, the government of the time, with its oligarchic liberal ideology, tackled public health problems by means of health campaigns aimed at combating epidemics, in other words, after the diseases had already taken on large proportions. This model of intervention became known as campanhista and was conceived within a military vision in which the ends justified the means, and in which the use of force and authority were considered the preferred instruments of action (POLIGNANO, 2007).

[a]In the final report of the 8th National Health Conference, the only reference to health education is linked to the incorporation of popular health agents as paid staff, under the coordination of the local level of the Unified Health System, to work in health education and primary care (BRASIL, 1986b). The Organic Health Law does not explicitly refer to the term either, but it does emphasise promotion, protection and preventive activities, in which we could consider that health education is implicitly included (BRASIL, 1990). Although both texts are emphatic in their broad conceptualisation of health, the lack of explicit reference to health education reflects the difficulty it has in being considered as an instrument for guaranteeing better health conditions (ALBUQUERQUE; STOTZ, 2004).

Popular Education is not the only pedagogical project to value the diversity and heterogeneity of social groups, intercommunication between different actors, commitment to the subaltern classes, the initiatives of the students and the dialogue between popular and scientific knowledge. But for the Brazilian health sector, the historical participation in the Popular Education movement was remarkable in the creation of a movement of professionals seeking to break with the authoritarian and standardising tradition of the relationship between health services and the population. Despite a certain crisis in the concept of Popular Education in new times, it is this concept that has served to identify and instrumentalise the diversity of emerging practices. In these experiences, the various methodological aspects valued are articulated in a peculiar way, different from what happens on other continents. There is an innovative and pioneering element in the Brazilian and Latin American experiences of Health Education that has been recognised internationally (VASCONCELOS, 2001).

Since primary care is the place where health education actions should be developed as a priority, and the Family Health Programme (PSF) is currently the main strategy for "reorienting the care model based on primary care" (BRASIL, 1997), it can be considered a favourable environment for the development of popular health education. National management bodies emphasise the importance of educational activities within the scope of the PSF, although no proposals have been developed for their funding, nor specific policies for the development of actions or even those aimed at training professionals (ALBUQUERQUE; STOTZ, 2004).

The PSF is being seen as an innovative model, based on a new social and cultural ethic, materialising the idea of health promotion, with a view to improving the quality of life of the Brazilian people. However, its sustainability requires the continuous establishment of intersectoral partnerships, articulating interdisciplinary actions of care, prevention and health promotion (SOUSA, 2004).

The concept of health education is anchored in the concept of health promotion, which deals with processes that involve the participation of the entire population in the context of their daily lives and not just people at risk of falling ill. This notion is based on the concept of health as a positive and dynamic state of well-being that integrates physical and mental (absence of disease), environmental, personal and social aspects (MACHADO et al, 2007).

Educating for health means going beyond curative care and prioritising preventive and promotional interventions. In this way, the development of educational practices within the scope of the PSF, whether in conventional spaces, such as educational groups, or in informal spaces, such as medical consultations at families' homes during home visits, expresses the assimilation of the principle of comprehensiveness by family health teams (ALVES, 2005).

The definition of a municipal health education policy, especially if it is based on the principles of popular education, would have the important role of inducing new practices in health services, fostering an appreciation of popular and user knowledge, showing professionals the educational nature of health actions, facilitating the participation of important social actors in the community in the process of building health (ALBUQUERQUE; STOTZ, 2004).

It is understood that the objectives of Health Education are to develop in people a sense of responsibility for their own health and the health of the community to which they belong, and the ability to participate in community life in a constructive way. It is therefore necessary to really evaluate these objectives and whether they are actually bringing about change in people's lives (OLIVEIRA; GONÇALVES, 2004).

The construction of knowledge based on reflections on the praxis of health education points to the need to implement a health education process involving the community through a participatory process that allows for critical reflection on reality and the determining factors of healthy living. Health education as a political and pedagogical process requires the development of critical and reflective thinking, allowing reality to be unveiled and transformative actions to be proposed that lead to the individual's autonomy and emancipation as a historical and social subject capable of proposing and having a say in health decisions to care for themselves, their family and the community (MACHADO et al, 2007).

Health education is a dynamic process that aims to empower individuals and/or groups in order to improve the population's health conditions. In this process, the population has the option of accepting or rejecting new information, and may or may not adopt new behaviours in the face of health problems. It is not enough just to follow recommended rules on how to be healthier and avoid illnesses, but rather to carry out health education in a process that stimulates dialogue, enquiry, reflection, questioning and shared action (MARTINS et al, 2007).

When analysing health education in services, another aspect of health practice is even more overlooked: the fact that every health action is an educational action. The promotion-prevention-cure-rehabilitation process is also a pedagogical process, in the sense that both the health professional and the client-user learn and teach. These concepts can effectively change the form and results of health work, transforming patients into citizens, co-participants in the process of building health (ALBUQUERQUE; STOTZ, 2004).

The educational dialogue between health authorities vested with educational and informational functions and the population becomes a mere discourse if it is not accompanied by a movement to strengthen, empower, economically, politically, socially and culturally subordinate individuals and groups (LEFÈVRE; LEFÈVRE, 2004).

It is precisely from the realisation of the ineffectiveness of education in bringing about changes in behaviour and practices in health education that the gap between discourse and pedagogical practice in health is established. Pedagogical practice remains stuck to the same principles, while the discourse of health education begins to appropriate new theoretical references that go beyond the deterministic notion between instituted knowledge and health practice. As a result, the theoretical discussion on health education has taken on new contours. In order to accompany it, it is necessary to understand the different axioms that have guided its development (GAZZINELLI et al, 2005).

Brazil is going through a period of demographic and epidemiological transition and it can be seen that the results presented here are in line with the proposed health strategies for this population group, as they showed that both for the prevalence rates in the sample in general and in the two regions studied, the elderly have always been more advised about the need to keep active and to carry out physical activity, as a health maintenance and prevention strategy (HIRVENSALO et al, 2003).

Freire (1997) emphasises that teaching is something profound and dynamic; therefore, "social and political solidarity" becomes essential in order to avoid elitist and authoritarian teaching, such as having exclusive control of "articulated knowledge". According to this author, educating is not merely transferring knowledge, but raising awareness and bearing witness to life, otherwise it won't be effective. The autonomy, dignity and identity of the learner, in this case the community and its subjects, must be respected, otherwise teaching will become "inauthentic, empty and inoperative verbiage" (BESEN et al, 2007).

Older people want to and can remain active and independent for as long as possible, if they are given the right support. The elderly are potentially at risk not just because they have grown old, but because the ageing process makes them more vulnerable to disability, largely as a result of adverse conditions in the physical or social environment, or affective issues. Adequate support is therefore needed for both the elderly and their carers (VERAS; CALDAS, 2004).

Extending life is an aspiration of every society. However, it can only be considered a real achievement to the extent that quality is added to the additional years of life. Therefore, any policy aimed at the elderly must take into account functional capacity, the need for autonomy, participation, care and self-satisfaction. It must also open up the possibility of acting in a variety of social contexts and developing new meanings for life in old age. And it should fundamentally encourage prevention, care and comprehensive health care (VERAS, 2009).

Programmes to encourage physical activity for this population are still scarce and little explored in health promotion environments, thus requiring greater attention from managers, health care, health education programmes and society itself. Few programmes to encourage physical activity have been developed in Brazil. However, the few initiatives have brought progress in this area (FRANCHI; JUNIOR, 2005).

The facts and evidence point to the urgent need for changes in care for the elderly population. Current models are proving to be inefficient and costly. Thus, new planning and management methods are needed, because the provision of care requires creative and innovative structures, with proposals for differentiated actions, so that the system gains efficiency and the elderly can fully enjoy the years provided by advances in science (LIMA; VERAS, 2003).

2.3 HEALTH LITERACY

The United Nations Educational, Scientific and Cultural Organisation - UNESCO (2005a) definition of literacy emphasises the context and use of literacy, conceived as the ability to identify, understand, interpret, create, communicate and assimilate, using printed and written materials associated with diverse contexts. Literacy involves a continuum of learning that enables individuals to achieve their goals, develop their knowledge and potential and participate fully in their community and society at large.

For UNESCO (2009), no definition of literacy can be permanent, above all because it should be taken as a process, the entry point to basic education and a means that leads to lifelong learning, and not as an end point. This conception is related to the pragmatic issues of language learning, and is configured as an instrument aimed at empowering people.

Paulo Freire (2005) also sees literacy as a process that allows connections to be made between the world in which a person lives and the written word; and from these connections, meanings and constructions of knowledge are born: "In a way, however, we can go further and say that reading the word is not only preceded by reading the world, but by a certain way of 'writing' or 'rewriting' it, that is, transforming it through our conscious practice. This dynamic movement is one of the central aspects of the literacy process".

The concept of health literacy is currently understood as integrating various levels of empowerment to make appropriate health choices such as choosing the health unit or service where to seek therapeutic help, adopting healthy lifestyles, or taking an active role in relation to the social determinants of health (NUTBEAM, 2000; RATZAN; PARKER, 2000).

Soares (2008; 2006) considers the strict meaning of the term literacy: "to literate is to make the individual capable of reading and writing". Different approaches to health literacy have been proposed. These include the functional and interactive approaches. Functional health literacy refers to mastering information about health risks and using health services. The interactive approach, on the other hand, involves personal skills that enable people and communities to expand their capacity to act independently (PASKULIN et al, 2011).

According to Nutbeam (2000), there are three types or levels of literacy: functional (or basic), interactive (communicational) and critical. This division makes it possible to see literacy in terms of the increasing autonomy and empowerment of individuals. "Functional/basic literacy: sufficient skills to read and write to enable effective functioning in everyday activities, broadly compatible with the definition of health literacy mentioned above; Interactive/communicative literacy: more advanced cognitive and literacy skills which, together with social skills, can be used to participate in day-to-day activities, to extract information and meaning from different forms of communication and apply this new information; Critical literacy: more advanced cognitive skills which, together with social skills, can be applied to critically analyse information and use this information to exercise greater control over life events and situations."

It should be noted that some population groups can be considered marginalised in terms of health literacy, such as the elderly, those with low levels of education and low incomes (CUTILLI, 2007). In Brazil, the challenge is greater when compared to other countries, despite the increase in life expectancy, the majority of elderly people live in unfavourable conditions, with low socioeconomic status, low schooling and a high prevalence of chronic diseases (ALLONI; PELÁEZ, 2003; LIMA; BARRETO; GIATTI, 2003). This phenomenon generates an impact and new demands on health services, leading to the need to (re)organise care models to meet the health needs of this population group (PASKULIN et al, 2011).

Brazil today is a "young country with grey hair". Every year 650,000 new elderly people are added to the Brazilian population, most of them with chronic diseases and some with functional limitations. In less than 40 years, Brazil has gone from a mortality scenario typical of a young population to a scenario of complex and costly illnesses, typical of long-lived countries, characterised by chronic and multiple diseases that last for years, requiring constant care, continuous medication and periodic examinations. The number of elderly people in Brazil rose from 3 million in 1960 to 7 million in 1975 and 20 million in 2008 - an increase of almost 700% in less than 50 years. As a result, age-related illnesses have become more prevalent in society as a whole (VERAS, 2009).

Population ageing is a fact of life that requires the development of programmes and actions capable of promoting health in old age, with a view to active and participatory ageing. According to Queiroz and Papaléo (2007), among all the programmes aimed at the elderly, aspects relating to sociability and education should take precedence in promoting healthy ageing. In this sense, understanding that social interaction and access to education inevitably depend on interlocutive processes that take place in the space of language production, it is worth highlighting the roles that reading and writing can play in the ageing process.

The *Offshore Installation Manager* (OIM), *Agency for Healthcare Research and Quality* (AHRQ) and *American Medical Association Ad Hoc Committee on Health Literacy* (AMA) have observed that large segments of the American population, such as half of all adults, lack the health literacy necessary to function properly in a healthcare environment. They would not, for example, be able to reliably and consistently determine the appropriate dose of cold medicine for a child, nor would they be able to read and understand informed consent documents (RUDD; KIRSCH, 2003; PAASCHE; TAYLOR; BRANCATI, 2003). Individuals with limited literacy come from all segments of society, and most are white, Native Americans (WEISS, 2004).

Communication theory distinguishes between different levels of information effectiveness (DERVIN, 2005). According to Thiede and Mcintyre (2008), the level at which health information becomes effective and empowers people in their choices regarding opportunities to use health services depends on a wide range of determinants. The effectiveness of information can be influenced by various characteristics on the recipient's side, such as their socioeconomic status, but it also depends on the socio-cultural relationship between the actors who are exchanging the information.

In fact, health communication includes messages that can have very different purposes, such as: promoting health and educating for health, avoiding risks and helping to deal with threats to health; preventing diseases; suggesting and recommending changes in behaviour; recommending screening tests; informing about health and diseases; informing about medical tests that need to be carried out and their results; prescribing medicines; recommending preventive measures and self-care activities for sick individuals (TEIXEIRA, 2004).

As for health systems, Rudd et al (2005) discuss that they rely on written texts to transmit various instructions, but that the readability of such texts often exceeds the users' ability to read. The authors also comment that there can be a dissonance between the actions of the health system and people's actual literacy skills, and exemplify this with health campaigns, which often require knowledge of complex concepts such as risk and probability (PASSAMAI et al, 2012).

In 2003, UNESCO coordinated the Action Plan for the Decade of Literacy 2003-2012, established at the 56ª session of the United Nations (UN) Assembly in 2001 (RICHMOND; ROBINSON; SACHS, 2009). This plan was guided by the goals of the World Education Forum, held in Dakar, Senegal, in 2000. These goals focused, among other important points, on reducing illiteracy by 50 per cent, as well as eliminating gender disparities in access to quality basic education and lifelong learning opportunities. Thus, promoting literacy among young people and adults and overcoming illiteracy in Brazil is seen as a challenge that is still far from being met in the country (UNESCO, 2008).

Client recall refers to the patient's ability to remember information and instructions received during a consultation. This recall involves information retained in both long-term and short-term memory and is also fundamental for adherence to treatment. A study cited by the authors points out that 80 per cent of medical information presented during a consultation is immediately forgotten and approximately half of the information recalled is incorrect (KESSELS, 2003).

The use of an instrument that assesses health literacy for employment in Brazil can provide support for planning care for the elderly population, since it is important to identify aspects relating to their health literacy so that professionals are able to promote health education to this population group, according to their own characteristics (PASKULIN et al, 2011).

Examples of these instruments are: a) Rapid Estimate of Adult Literacy in Medicine (REALM) 37, which measures only numerical skills, using questions about food portion sizes; b) Wide Range Achievement Test, third edition (WRAT-3) (WILKINSON, 1993) c) Short Test of Functional Health Literacy (STOFHLA) (DAVIS et al, 1998), which is a shortened version of the Test of Functional Health Literacy (TOFHLA) (PARKER et al, 1995). While the latter measures reading comprehension and numeracy (numeracy*) -

implying an average completion time of 22 minutes - the STOFHLA only assesses reading comprehension (with an average completion time of 7 minutes; d) Newest Vital Sign (NVS). This is a quick-to-use health literacy measurement tool with only six items, which involves interpreting written and numerical information. Before answering each item, the person has to read an information leaflet with nutritional information (WEISS et al, 2005). The instrument was designed to be applied in a primary care setting. As already mentioned, there is a Portuguese version with some known psychometric properties (LUIS; LOUREIRO, 2008).

Studies were carried out to produce a health literacy tool in Portuguese and during planning it was realised that it would have the same problem as the Spanish translation of REALM because Portuguese also has transparent orthography with high grapheme-phoneme correspondences. The author's hypothesis is that SAHLSA could be translated into Portuguese without any structural changes and with minimal semantic adjustments (APOLINÁRIO et al, 2012).

The SAHLSA instrument was then translated from Spanish into Portuguese, where it was carried out independently by two bilingual health professionals who were not involved in the study. The translators were informed about the purpose of the study and the target population. To ensure concept equivalence, the translated versions of the instrument were analysed by four members of the research team to resolve any discrepancies and a consensus version was drawn up. This version was pre-tested on a pilot sample of 20 older adults to identify idiomatic and cultural issues. The results were satisfactory, with no changes needed to the medical terms. Only one word association was replaced to improve clarity, states the study by Apolinário et al (2012).

In a second step, the back translation from Brazilian Portuguese into Spanish was carried out by a professional translator who was unaware of the study's objectives and did not take part in any of the previous stages of the study. The equivalence assessment showed satisfactory results; 99 per cent of the back translation showed semantic agreement with the SAHLSA. The resulting instrument was then named the Breve de Avaliação da Saúde de Alfabetização para Adultos de língua Português (SAHLPA).

Apolinário et al (2012) describes that the administration of the SAHLPA was similar to that of the SAHLSA. Laminated flash cards were used, each with a medical term printed in bold at the top and two association words at the bottom. One of the words was significantly associated with the medical term and the other was not. Respondents were shown a flash card one at a time and asked to read aloud the medical term in bold. The interviewer then read out the two association words and asked the interviewee which one was significantly associated with the medical term. The aim of the association questions was to assess comprehension, so the interviewees were instructed not to guess and say "I don't know" if they didn't know the correct association. The answer was considered correct only when the interviewee pronounced the medical term correctly and made the correct association. One point was scored for each correct item, with a maximum score of 50. User instructions and laminated card games are available on request from the corresponding author.

No formal agreement has yet been reached on the criteria to be used to select the most appropriate measure of health literacy for different groups (POWERS; TRINH; BOSWORTH, 2010). Measurement selection can be particularly important in healthcare settings, where the importance of patient understanding of health management is essential. The issue of measurement selection is especially important with older adults, where substantial variation in educational attainment and interactions with healthcare across the lifespan raises concerns about the duration and complexity of health literacy tools (FEDERMAN et al, 2009). The S-TOFHLA can address length and complexity, but few studies have evaluated the performance of alternative tools such as the SF-realm and the NVS in older populations (MANCUSO, 2009). Kirk et al (2011) show that the evaluation of Common tools are an essential step towards enabling rigorous primary care research focussed on the role of health literacy in shaping the experiences and clinical outcomes of older adults.

Special attention should be paid to the language of health-related texts, since even a high level of education may not be enough to understand the meaning of medical and technical language. Health-related terms can be more difficult than those required for basic reading and comprehension skills in other texts (AMA, 1999). This complexity, combined with the lack of a consensus on the definition of health literacy, generates a demand for criteria to assess people's level of literacy (OZDEMIR et al, 2010; BARBER et al, 2009; ISHIKAWA; YANO, 2008; BAKER; 2006; PARKER et al, 1995).

3 METHODOLOGY

A validated Brief Assessment of Health Literacy for Portuguese-Speaking Adults (SAHLPA) instrument was used, consisting of 50 items that assessed the individual's ability to correctly pronounce and understand common medical terms, thus screening for inadequate health literacy, as this situation is associated with lower use of preventive services, poor self-management of chronic diseases, low adherence to medication, increased hospitalisation and higher mortality rates (APOLINÁRIO et al, 2012).

The sample consisted of 100 elderly residents of the city of Oeiras, a Brazilian municipality in the state of Piauí, located more precisely in the smallest region of south-eastern Piauí, in the microregion of Picos. As the first capital, it is strategically located in the centre of the state, with an estimated population of 36,266 in 2014 (IBGE, 2014). The elderly attended the Basic Health Units and/or the Clube da Melhor Idade with the following inclusion criteria: age > 60 years, hypertensive and/or diabetic, self-reported ability to read and speak Portuguese; no diagnosis of dementia; no visual impairment or hearing problems that would not allow adequate interaction with the interviewers. Individuals who self-reported being illiterate, i.e. were unable to read at all, were excluded from the study, as the health literacy test will be purposeless. All subjects were informed about the purpose and procedures of the study. An informed consent was obtained before the interview.

The questionnaire was administered in between each activity at the Clube da Melhor Idade and at other times the survey was carried out at the homes of elderly people attending the Basic Health Units. The elderly were approached individually and invited to answer the questionnaire. After accepting the invitation, they read the slides and answered the questions while the researcher transcribed each participant's answers.

4 RESULTS AND DISCUSSION

Based on the analysis of the answers to the questionnaires, it can be said that, in terms of the general characterisation of the sample, there was a predominance of females, representing 76%. Of the 100 elderly people interviewed, 16% were aged between 60 and 64, 20% were aged between 65 and 69 and 31% were aged between 70 and 74, 20% were aged between 75 and 79 and 8% were aged between 80 and 84, the other 5% were aged 85 or over. The minimum age was 60 and the maximum 86, with an average age of 72, as can be seen in Table 1.

TABLE 1- DISTRIBUTION OF THE SAMPLE ACCORDING TO AGE (IN YEARS)- 2014.

AGE (YEARS)	n	%
60 a 64	16	16
65 a 69	20	20
70 a 74	31	31
75 a 79	20	20
80 a 84	8	8
85 or more	5	5
TOTAL	100	100

Source: The author

Estimates suggest that over the next 20 years the number of elderly people in Brazil is likely to exceed 30 million, making up almost 13% of the population (FRANK et al, 2007). These figures characterise a population of long-lived individuals, corroborating the growth of the elderly population in Brazil and also showing an improvement in life expectancy and the need for more specific policies and actions in this area.

and the need for more policies and specific actions to promote health, aimed at an active and participative public.

In this respect, the data from this research coincides with the study by Veras (2009), which shows the increase in the number of elderly people in the country and consequently the increase in life expectancy, where ageing is a fact that needs attention. Palloni and Peláez (2003) show that population ageing is a global phenomenon that does not occur in the same way in all countries. In developed countries, the increase in the elderly population has occurred gradually, while in developing countries, the demographic transition has occurred rapidly and progressively.

Another important finding among the participants is that they suffer from hypertension (74 per cent), diabetes and hypertension simultaneously (21 per cent) and only diabetes (5 per cent), according to figure 1.

FIGURE 1- DISTRIBUTION OF ELDERLY PEOPLE BY PATHOLOGY

Source: The author

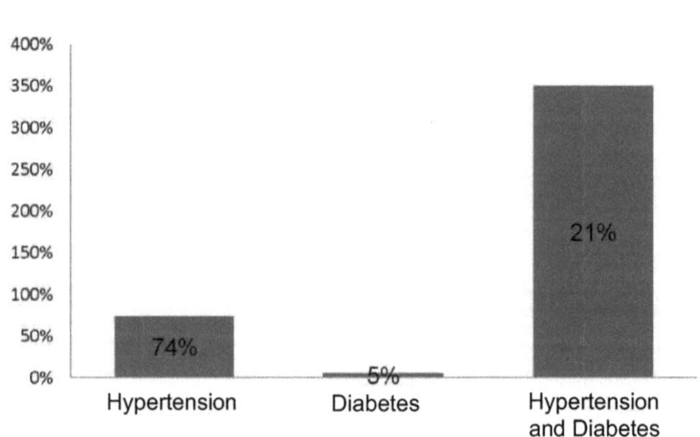

The majority, 74 per cent of the elderly, have hypertension, which is higher than the Brazilian Heart Society (2010), which states that in Brazil its prevalence is between 22.3 and 43.9 per cent, with an average of 32.5 per cent, affecting more than 50 per cent of elderly individuals aged between 60 and 69 and 75 per cent of those aged over 70 (SBC, 2010).

Five per cent of the sample has diabetes and the prevalence of the disease in Brazil, according to data from the 2011 Surveillance of Risk and Protective Factors for Chronic Diseases by Telephone Survey (Vigitel), shows that the prevalence of self-reported diabetes in the population over 18 increased from 5.3 per cent to 5.6 per cent between 2006 and 2011. Another 21 per cent of the elderly interviewed have both hypertension and diabetes, and it can be seen that hypertension is around twice as frequent among diabetic patients when compared to the general population, says the Guide to Adult Health Care: Hypertension and Diabetes (2006).

When it comes to the questions on the test applied in the study, it is noteworthy that the interviewees got an average of only 34 out of 50 questions right, much lower than the 43 points that must be achieved in order to qualify for an adequate level of health literacy, the minimum score was 23 points and the maximum was 48 points, the majority of the elderly got it wrong or didn't know the meaning of everyday scientific terms such as: constipation, colitis and jaundice, for example. Despite the fact that all the participants in the study had completed some level of schooling, 92% of the elderly who took the SAHLPA-50 questionnaire had inadequate health literacy, an average higher than that of the study carried out by Apolinário et al (2012), who found that 66% of the study sample had inadequate health literacy.

In the survey carried out by Lee et al in 2010, with 1,492 Taiwanese adults, but using the MHLS (a reading and maths instrument to assess health literacy in Mandarin Chinese or Standard Chinese) 69.7% of respondents had adequate health literacy, 16.6% marginal, and 13.7% inadequate. In general, the level of health literacy was lower among adults with older age, fewer years of formal schooling, lower family income, and who lived in less populated areas.

According to Neri (2007), 49% of Brazil's elderly population is considered functionally illiterate. Of this total, 23% say they can't read and write, 4% say they can only read and write their own name and 22% of the elderly find reading and writing difficult, either because of learning disabilities, health problems or both. In other words, a significant portion of the elderly population remains on the margins of today's graphocentric society, confirming the need to implement public policies that include literacy activities for this population. Since low literacy rates have been linked to adverse health outcomes, including hospitalisations, an increase in some chronic diseases and higher healthcare costs (SANCHEZ; CICONELLI, 2012).

This information coincides with the results of this study where there is a high rate of inadequate health literacy among the elderly, so attention and educational counselling for them should be prioritised. According to Perlow (2010), health literacy enables people to make appropriate decisions and understand their own health needs. It involves personal skills that enable people and communities to expand their capacity to act independently (PASKULIN et al, 2011).

In this sense, it is important to emphasise the role of health and education professionals in this scenario to make proposals capable of promoting healthy ageing and inserting the elderly into today's society (TORQUATO; MASSI; SANTANA, 2011). Actions offered by the government, which offer possibilities for health literacy, qualifying the ability of each elderly person to read and understand a text, increasing their power of discussion and enabling them to seek their rights in society.

It is plausible to take into account that most of the elderly have limited health literacy, which indicates that the difficulties range from economic to social and historical issues. The participants in this study don't seem to have had much of a connection between writing developed at school and writing in other contexts. It's as if writing had been taught simply to read and not to understand and assimilate a text with experience. As a result, they are deprived of health and education and have a poor quality of life.

Further studies with a representative sample are needed to validate the results and the extent of the problem is complicated to assess because inter-rater reliability has never been tested, but even so the SAHLPA-50 is a valid and reliable instrument and an essential step for health literacy research in Brazil and even for other Portuguese-speaking countries (APOLINÁRIO et al, 2012).

Health literacy is therefore seen as a fundamental skill so that, on a day-to-day basis, each individual can make the best health decisions, take control of their health and be an active and responsible partner (REIS, 2010).

5. FINAL CONSIDERATIONS

The elderly population has been increasing, as the group surveyed shows, with a life expectancy of 72 years, and this emphasises the need for a more interactive and practical health education process. Society needs to review its political and educational projects as a way of promoting ageing with quality of life and cultivating new habits so that the elderly can achieve the possibility of self-realisation and independence.

In this research, all the elderly people studied were fully capable of understanding and absorbing knowledge. It was possible to investigate that the level of health literacy is very low, i.e. an unsatisfactory level, such conditions depend on a whole change in the system in which we live. The methodological procedures used proved to be effective because they made it possible to investigate levels of health literacy, and so this article was able to achieve its initial objectives.

Consideration should be given to the view that older people have of the benefits that writing and reading can bring to successful ageing. When we read and write we are exercising our cognition or even a motor skill of great significance in the social context, since these are practices that enable their access to health, education, leisure and work. It is therefore necessary to emphasise the increase in reading and writing practices with the elderly because this goes far beyond a mere cognitive notion.

The results found in this study suggest that health professionals and society as a whole should seek to develop health literacy practices, introducing technical and scientific terms to the elderly, as well as promoting experience with science, where such activities should reduce access difficulties, associating health promotion and prevention with educational work, and consequently the achievement of life rights.

Having said this, we can say that there is great expectation in our society, since the development of SALPHA-50 has already leveraged goals and planning with regard to health literacy and will now encourage more studies to improve inadequate health literacy and minimise the negative impacts in the whole area of health.

REFERENCES

ALBUQUERQUE, P. C.; STOTZ, E. N. Popular education in primary care: in search of comprehensive health care, **Interface - Comunic., Saúde, Educ.**, v.8, p.259-74, mar/ago, 2004.

ALVES V. S. A health education model for the Family Health Programme: towards comprehensive health care and model reorientation, **Interface - Comunic., Saúde, Educ.**, v.9, n.16, p.39-52, set.2004/fev, 2005.

AKERMAN M, MENDES R, BÓGUS C.M. Is it possible to evaluate an ethical imperative? **Ciência e Saúde Coletiva**, v.11, p.605-13, July/September, 2004.

AMERICAN MEDICAL ASSOCIATION AD HOC COMMITTEE ON HEALTH LITERACY (AMA). Health literacy: report of the council on scientific affairs. **JAMA**, v.281, p.552-7, 1999.

ANDRADE L.O. M. **SUS passo a passo: normas, gestão e financiamento**. São Paulo: Hucitec, 2001.

APOLINÁRIO et al. **Short Health Literacy Assessment for Portuguese-speaking Adults**. Geriatrics Department. Faculty of Medicine (FM). University of São Paulo (USP). São Paulo, SP, Brazil[II] Department of Neurology. FM-USP.São Paulo, SP, Brazil[m] School of Public Health. University of Michigan.Ann Arbor, MI, USA, 2012.

ADULT HEALTH CARE: HYPERTENSION AND DIABETES. Belo Horizonte: SAS/MG, MINAS GERAIS. **State Department of Health**, 2006.

BAKER D.W. The meaning and the measure of health literacy. **J. Gen. Intern. Med.**, v.21, p.878-83, 2006.

BAKER et al. Health literacy, cognitive abilities, and mortality among elderly persons. **J Gen Intern Med**, v.23, p.723-6, jun, 2008.

BARBER et al. Up to a quarter of the Australian population may have suboptimal health literacy depending upon the measurement tool: results from a population-based survey. **Health Promot**. Int., v.24, p.252-61, 2009.

BERNHARDT J.; BROWNFIELD E.; PARKER, R. - **Understanding health literacy**. In SCHWARTZBERG, J.; VANGEEST, J.; WANG, C., ed. lit.Understanding health literacy: implications for medicine and public health.
Chicago: AMA Press, p.13-16, 2005.

BESEN et al. The Family Health Strategy as an Object of Health Education. **Saúde e Sociedade**, v.16, p.57-68, jan-abr, 2007.

BRASIL. **Saúde da família: uma estratégia para a reorientação do modelo assistencial**. Brasília: Ministry of Health, 1997.

BRAZIL. **Ministry of Health. Health Policy Secretariat**, Health Promotion Project. Declarations of health promotion conferences, Brasilia, 2001.

BRAZIL. Ministry of Health. Health Surveillance Secretariat. Secretariat for Strategic and Participatory Management. **Vigitel-Brasil 2011:** surveillance of risk and protective factors for chronic diseases by telephone survey. Brasília, 2012.

BUSS P. **Priority approaches in public health.** In: Pan American Health Organisation. Challenges for public health education, sectoral reform and essential public health functions. Washington: OPS. p.7-26, 2000.

BUSS P. **An introduction to the concept of health promotion**. In: Czeresnia D, Freitas CM, organisers. Health promotion: concepts, reflections, trends. Rio de Janeiro: Fiocruz. p.15-38, 2003.

BYDLOWSKI C. R., PEREIRA I. M.T. B., WESTPHAL M. F. Health Promotion. Why yes and why not yet! **Saúde e Sociedade**, v.13, p.14-24, jan-abr, 2004.

CAMPOS et al. Avaliação de política nacional de promoção da saúde. **Ciência & Saúde Coletiva**, v. 9, p.745-749, 2004.

CARVALHO R.S. **Saúde coletiva e promoção á saúde: uma reflexão sobre os temas do sujeito e da mudança**.2002.[thesis]. Campinas (SP): Postgraduate Programme in Medical Sciences/Unicamp, 2002.

CARVALHO A. C. Dualism and alienation. **Scientific American Brasil**, n.12, p.29, May 2003.

CARVALHO S. R. As contradições da promoção à saúde em relação à produção de sujeitos e a mudança social. **Ciência & Saúde Coletiva**, v.9, p. 669-678, 2004.

CUTILLI C. C. Health literacy in geriatric patients: An integrative review of the literature. **Orthop Nurs**, v.26, p.43-8, 2007.

CZERESNIA D**. The concept of health and the difference between prevention and promotion.** In: Czeresnia D, Freitas CM, organisers. Health promotion: concepts, reflections, trends. Rio de Janeiro: Fiocruz;.

p.39- 53, 2003.

DERVIN B. Libraries reaching out with health information to vulnerable populations: guidance from research on information seeking and use. **J Med Libr Assoc.**, v.93, p.74-80, 2005.

FEDERMAN et. al. Health literacy and cognitive performance in older adults. **J Am Geriatric Soc.**, v.57, p.1475-80, 2009.

FRANCHI K.M.B.; JUNIOR R.M.M. Physical Activity: a necessity for a good heath in old age. **Brazilian Journal in Heath Promotion**, v.18, p.152-156, 2005.

FRANK et al. The assessment of functional capacity: Rethinking care for the elderly in Community Health. **Interdisciplinary Studies in Ageing**, 2007.

FREIRE, P. **Pedagogia da autonomia: saberes necessárias à pratica educativa**. 5. ed. São Paulo: Paz e Terra, 1997.

FREIRE P. **A importância do ato de ler - em três artigos que se completam**, São Paulo: Cortez, 2005.

GAZZINELLI et al. Health education: knowledge, social representations and experiences of the disease. **Cad. Saúde Pública,** Rio de Janeiro, v.21, p.200-206, jan-feb, 2005.

GIRONDI J, NOTHAFT S, MALLMANN F. A metodologia problematizadora utilizada pelo enfermeiro na educação sexual de adolescentes. **Cogitare Enferm.**, v.11, p.161-5, May/Aug. 2006.

HEIDMANN et. al. Health promotion: historical trajectory of its conceptions. **Texto Contexto Enferm**, Florianópolis, v.15, p.352-8, Apr-Jun. 2006.

HIRVENSALO et al. The effect of advice by health care professionals on increasing physical activity of older people. **Scand J Med Sci Sports**, v. 13, p.231-6, 2003.

BRAZILIAN INSTITUTE OF GEOGRAPHY AND STATISTICS (IBGE). **Brazilian population according to the census**, 2014. Available at <http: www.diabetes.org.br>. Accessed on 01 December 2014.

INSTITUTE OF MEDICINE. Health Literacy: a prescription to end the confusion. Washington DC: **National Academic Press**, 2004.

ISHIKAWA H.; YANO E. Patient health literacy and participation in the health-care process. **Health Expect**. v.11, p.113-22, 2008.

KWAMOTO E. E. **Enfermagem comunitária.** São Paulo: EPU, 1995.

KELLY, HAIDET. Physician overestimation of patient literacy: A potential source of patient health disparities. **Educ Couns**, v. 66, p.119- 22., 2007.

KESSELS R. P. Patients' memory for medical information. **Soc Med.**, v.96 , p.219-22, 2003.

KIRK et al. Health literacy test performance among older adults with diabetes. **J Gen Intern Med**, v.27, p.534-40, May 2012.

LABONTE R. **Estrategias para la promoción de la salud en la comunidad**. In: PANAMERICAN HEALTH ORGANISATION. Health promotion: an anthology. Washington: PAHO, p. 153-65. (Scientific publication, 557), 1996.

LABONTE R. **Community empowerment and leisure**. J. Leisurability, v.23, n.1, 1996b. Available at <http://www.lin.ca/resource/html/Vol23/v23n1a2.htm>. Accessed on: 02 October 2014.

LALONDE M. **A new perspective on the health of Canadians**. Ottawa: Health and Welfare, 1974.

LEE et al. Health literacy, health status, and healthcare utilisation of Taiwanese adults: results from a national survey. **BMC Public Health.** Taiwan, v.10, n. 614, p.4, 2010.

LEFEVRE, F.; LEFEVRE, A. M. C. **Promoção de saúde, a negação da negação**. Rio de Janeiro: Vieira & Lent, 2004.

LEVY et al. **Health education: history, concepts and proposals.** Brasília (DF) 2003; [on line]. Available at: <http:www.datasus.gov.br/cns.>Accessed on: 20 Oct. 2014.

LIMA-COSTA M. F, VERAS R. P. Saúde pública e envelhecimento. **Cad Saude Publica**, 2003.

LUIS L.F.S, LOUREIRO I. **Health literacy and food.** In Jorge Bonito. Health education in the 21st century - theories, models and practices. CIEP - Centre for Research in Education and Psychology, 2 008.

MACHADO et al. Integrality, health training, health education and SUS proposals - a conceptual review. **Ciência & Saúde Coletiva**, v. 12, p.335-342, 2007.

MACIEL M.E.D. **A educação em saúde na concepção do agentes comunitários de saúde de Fátima do Sul-MS** [monografia].Campo Grande (MS):Universidade Federal de Mato Grosso do Sul, 2008.

MACIEL M.E. D. EDUCAÇÃO EM SAÚDE: CONCEITOS E PROPÓSITOS. **Cogitare Enferm**, v.14, p.773-6, Oct/Dec. 2009.

MANAFO WONG. Health literacy programmes for older adults: a systematic literature review. **Health Education Research**, v.27, p.947-960, 2012.

MANCUSO J.M. Assessment and measurement of health literacy: na integrative review of the literature. **Nurs Health Sci.**, v.11, p.77-89, 2 009.

MARTINS et al. health education needs of carers of elderly people at home. **Texto Contexto Enferm**, Florianópolis, v.16, p. 254-62, abr-jun. 2007.

MINISTRY OF HEALTH (BR). **Health promotion charters.** Brasília: The Ministry, 2002.

NERI A. L. **Idosos no Brasil: Vivências, desafios e expectativas na terceira idade**. São Paulo, SP: Perseu Abramo Foundation, 2007.

NUTBEAM D. Health literacy as a public health goal: a challenge for contemporary health education and communication strategies into the 21st century. **Health Promotion International**. v.15, p.259-67, sep. 2000.

OLIVEIRA H. M., GONÇALVES M. J. F. EDUCAÇÃO EM SAÚDE: uma experiência transformadora. **Rev Bras Enferm**, Brasília (DF), v. 57, p.761-3, nov/dez. 2004.

OLIVEIRA D.L. The 'new' public health and health promotion through education: between tradition and innovation. **Ver Latino-am Enfermagem**, v.13, p.423-31, May-June. 2005.

UNITED NATIONS ORGANISATION FOR EDUCATION, SCIENCE AND CULTURE - UNESCO. **Youth and adult literacy in Brazil: lessons from practice. Brasilia**: UNESCO, 2008.

UNITED NATIONS ORGANISATION FOR EDUCATION, SCIENCE AND CULTURE - UNESCO. Education Sector. Division for the Coordination of

United Nations Priorities in Education. **The challenge of global literacy: a profile of youth and adult literacy halfway through the United Nations Decade for Literacy**, 2003-2012. Brasilia: UNESCO, 2009.

WORLD HEALTH ORGANISATION (OMS). **Ottawa Charter for Health Promotion. First International Conference on Health Promotion.** Ottawa, 21 November 1986 - WHO/HPR/HEP/95.1.Available at: <http://www.who.int/hpr/NPH/docs/ottawa_charter_hp.pdf.> Accessed on: 01 October 2014.

PAN AMERICAN HEALTH ORGANISATION - OPS. **Indicators for the municipal health movement.** Washington: PAHO, 1995.

OSVALDO S. The role of health literacy: empowering overweight people to control and reduce their weight burden.
Endocrinology, Diabetes & Obesity, vol. 4, jul/set, 2010.

OZDEMIR et al. Health literacy among adults: a study from Turkey. **Health Educ Res.**, v.25, p.464-77, 2010.
PAASCHE-ORLOW M. K, TAYLOR H. A, BRANCATI F. L. Readability standards for informed consent forms compared with actual reading. **N Engl J Med**, v.348, p.721-726, 2003.

PALLONI A, PELÁEZ M. **History and nature of the study.** In: Lebrão ML, Duarte YAO, organisers. SABE - Health, Well-being and Ageing - The SABE project in the municipality of São Paulo: an initial approach. Brasília: Pan American Health Organisation,. p. 13-32, 2003.

PARKER et al. THE TEST OF FUNCTIONAL HEALTH LITERACY IN ADULTS: A NEW INSTRUMENT FOR MEASURING PATIENTS' LITERACY SKILLS. **J. Gen. Intern. Med.**, v.10, p.537-41, 1995.

PARKER R.M, RATZAN S.C, LURIE N. Health literacy: a challenge for advancing high-quality health care policy. **Aff Health**, v.22, p. 147-53, 2003.

PASKULIN et al. Adaptation of an instrument that assesses health literacy in the elderly. **Acta Paul Enferm**, v.24, p.271-7, 2011.

PASSAMAI M et al. Functional health literacy: reflections and concepts on its impact on the interaction among users, professionals and the health system. **Interface - Comunic., Saude, Educ.**, v.16, p.301-14, apr./jun, 2012.

PERLOW E. Accessibility: global gateway to health literacy. **Health Promot Pract.**, v.11, p.123-31, 2010.

POLIGNANO M. V. **História das políticas de saúde no Brasil: uma pequena revisão**, 2007. Available at:<http://www.internatorural.medicina.ufmg.br/ saude_no_brasil.rtf.>Accessed on: 15 Oct. 2014.

POTVIN L, HADDAD S, FROHLICH K. L. **Beyond process and outcome evaluation: a comprehensive approach for evaluating health promotion programmes.** In: WHO. Europe evaluation in health promotion: principies and perspectives. Copenhagen (Denmark): WHO - Europe;. p. 45-62, 2001.

POWERS B.J, TRINH J.V, BOSWORTH H.B. Can this patient read and understand written health information? **JAMA**, v. 304, p.76-84, 2010.

QUEIROZ Z. P. V., PAPALÉO N.M. **Successful ageing: Biological, psychological and socio-cultural aspects. The importance of sociability and education.** In M. P. Papaléo Netto (Ed.), Tratado de Gerontologia (pp. 807- 816). São Paulo, SP: Atheneu, 2007.

RATZAN S. C, PARKER R. M. Health literacy. Current Bibliographies in Medicine, 2000-1. Bethesda, MD. **National Library of Medicine**, 2000. Available at:<http://www.nlm.nih.gov/archive/20061214/pubs/cbm/hliteracy.html. Accessed on: 02 October 2014.

RECIIS - **Revista Eletrônica de Comunicação Informação e Inovação em Saúde**. Rio de Janeiro, v.3, n.3, p.58-66, set., 2009.

REIS, L. A. S. B. **O conhecimento sobre o medicamento e a literacia em saúde**: Um estudo em adultos, utentes de farmácias do concelho de Lisboa.Thesis for the master's degree in health and development. Instituto de Higiene e Medicina Tropical Universidade Nova de Lisboa, v.1, p. 65, 2010.

REISI et. al. Relationship between health literacy, health status and healthy behaviours among the elderly in Isfahan. **J Health Syst Res**, v.7, p.1-12, 2011.

RICHMOND M.; ROBINSON C.; SACHS-ISRAEL M. **The global literacy challenge: a profile of youth and adult literacy at the halfway point of the United Nations Decade for Literacy**, 2003-2012. Paris: Unesco, 2009.

ROTHMAN et al. Patient understanding of food labels: the role of literacy and numeracy. **Am J Prev Med**, v.31, p.391-8, nov, 2006.

RUDD R, KIRSCH L, K. Yamamoto. Literacy in Health Settings: A Re-analysis of the NALS. American Public Health Association Annual Conference Session 4.182,1. Washington, DC. **American Public Health Association**, 2003.

RUDD et al. **Literacy demands in health care settings: the patient perspective**. In: SCHWARTZBERG, J.G.; VENGEEST, J.B.; WANG, C.C. (Orgs.). Understanding health literacy: implications for medicine and public health. United States: AMA. p.69-85, 2005.

SANCHEZ R.M, CICONELLI R.M. Concepts of access to health. **Rev Panam Salud Publica**, v.31, p.260-8, 2012.

SBC, BRAZILIAN SOCIETY OF CARDIOLOGY. **VI Brazilian Hypertension Guidelines**. Rio de Janeiro, 2010.

SCHALL V. T, STUCHINER M. Health education: new perspectives. **Cad. Saúde Pública**, v.2, p.4-5, 1999.

SÍCOLI J. L., NASCIMENTO P. R. Health promotion: concepts, principles and practice, **Interface - Comunic Saúde, Educ**, v.7, p.91- 112, 2003.

SIMONDS, S. Health education as social policy. **Health Education Monograph,** v.2, p. 1-25, 1974.

SOARES. **Letramento: a theme in three genres.** Belo Horizonte: Autêntica, 2006.

SOARES, M. **Alfabetização e letramento**. 5.ed. São Paulo: Contexto, 2008.

SOUSA M. F. **The Family Health Programme: a national vision**. In: Fernandes MEL, Dowbor TP, Kretzer MR, Gouveia I, Sucupira AC, Menezes L, Resegue R, organisers. AIDS: door-to-door prevention. São Paulo: Hucitec, v. 1, p. 41-5, 2004.

SUDORE R.L, YAFFE K, SATTERFIELD S, et al. limited literacy and mortality in the elderly: the health, aging, and body composition study. **J Gen Intern Med**, v.21, p.806-12, 2006.

TEERÃ: **Jam-e-Jam newspaper Cabinet**; [Updated 2012 01 July; cited 2012 01 July]. Jamejam online. Available at: <http://www.jamejamonline.ir/newstext.aspx?newsnum=100004064059.> Accessed on: 10 Oct. 2014.

TEHRANI-BANIHASHEMI et. al. Health in five provinces of the country and its determinants. **Advances in Medical Education Development**, v.1, p.1-9, 2007.

TEIXEIRA, J. Comunicação em saúde: relação técnicos de saúde - utentes. **Análise Psicológica**. v.22, n.3, p. 615-620, 2004.

THIEDE M, MCINTYRE D. Information, communication and equitable access to health care: a conceptual note. **Cad Saude Publica**, v.24, p.1168-73, 2008.

TORQUATO R., MASSI G., SANTANA A. P. Ageing and Literacy: Reading and Writing from the Perspective of People Over 60 Years of Age. **Psicologia: Reflexão e Crítica**, v.24, p. 89-98, 2011.

UNITED NATIONS EDUCATIONAL, SCIENTIFIC AND CULTURAL ORGANISATION - UNESCO. **Aspects of literacy assessment: topics and issues from the UNESCO expert meeting**. Paris: UNESCO, 2005a.

VASCONCELOS E. Educação popular como instrumento de reorientação das estratégias de controle das doenças infecciosas e parasitárias. **Cad Saúde Pública**, v.14, p.39-57, 1998.

VASCONCELOS E. M. Redefinindo as práticas de Saúde a partir de experiências de Educação Popular nos serviços de saúde. **Interface - Comunic, Saúde, Educ.** February, 2001.
VERAS R. P., CALDAS P. C. Promoting the health and citizenship of the elderly: the third age university movement. **Ciência & Saúde Coletiva**, v.9, p.423-432, 2004.

VERAS R. Ageing, demands, challenges and innovations. **Rev Saúde Pública**, v.43, p.548-54, 2009.

WEISS B. **Epidemiology of low educational attainment**. In: Schwartzberg J, VanGeest J, Wang C, eds Understanding Health Literacy: Implications for Medicine and Public Health. Chicago, Illinois: American Medical Association Press, 17-42, 2004.

WEISS et al. Quick assessment of literacy in primary care: the newest vital sign. **Ann Fam Med**, v.3, p.514-22, Nov-Dec. 2005.

WORLD HEALTH ORGANISATION. **Health promotion evaluation: recommendations to policymakers**. Copenhagen: European Working Group on Health Promotion Evaluation, 1998.

ZARCADOOLAS C, PLEASANT A, GREER D. Advancing health literacy. A framework for understanding and action. **San Francisco: John Wiley &**

Sons, 2006.

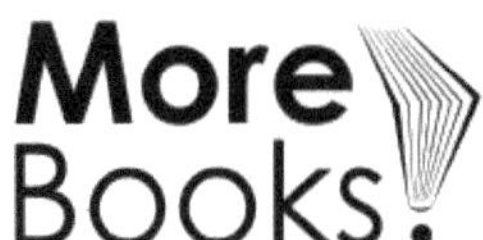

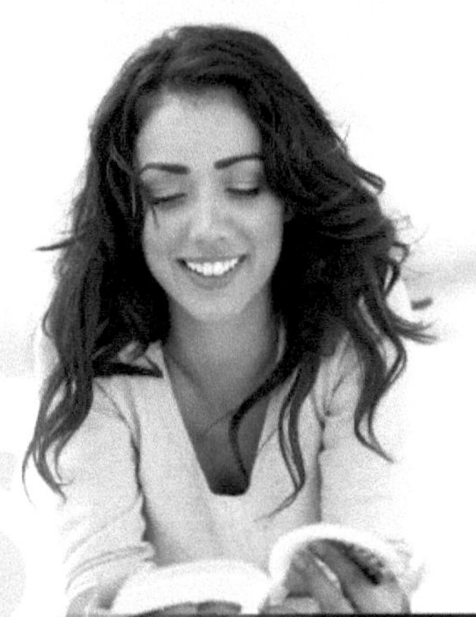

I want morebooks!

Buy your books fast and straightforward online - at one of world's fastest growing online book stores! Environmentally sound due to Print-on-Demand technologies.

Buy your books online at
www.morebooks.shop

Kaufen Sie Ihre Bücher schnell und unkompliziert online – auf einer der am schnellsten wachsenden Buchhandelsplattformen weltweit! Dank Print-On-Demand umwelt- und ressourcenschonend produziert.

Bücher schneller online kaufen
www.morebooks.shop

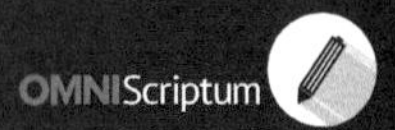

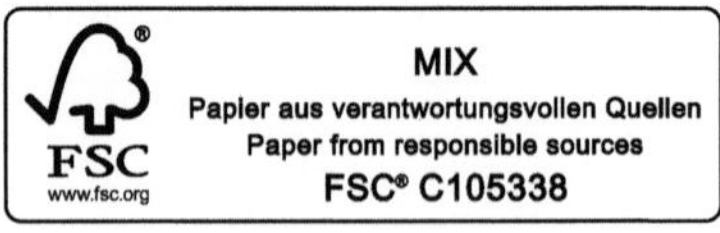

Printed by Books on Demand GmbH, Norderstedt / Germany